In The Shelter
Of
His Arms

In The Shelter Of His Arms

M. DIANNE ROSE

To order additional copies of this book, contact:
Xlibris Corporation
1-888-795-4274
www.Xlibris.com
Orders@Xlibris.com
120214

CONTENTS

DEDICATION

I WISH TO DEDICATE THIS BOOK, FIRST OF ALL, TO MY LORD AND SAVIOR, JESUS CHRIST. Without His help and inspiration, it would be impossible to write my story. Secondly, I want to thank my husband, Bob, who has been a constant help and source of encouragement. He has had faith in me and my desire to accomplish this work of love.

I also want to acknowledge the support of my children in writing my story. They have been my biggest fans, and I thank God for each one of them: Candee, Michael and Rhonda. They have seen me during my best days and my worst days, and they still love me. It is my constant prayer that I will be a living sacrifice of God's love and miraculous healing power.

I especially want to thank the wonderful medical doctors and nurses who used their knowledge and surgical expertise which were crucial in my recovery. The most recent surgical team at St. Louis University Hospital were wonderful angels of healing, as were the cancer specialists at Muskogee Regional Cancer Center.

I have been blessed with many good friends. I cannot forget to remember my employer and co-workers at Healthcare Solutions Group in Muskogee, Oklahoma. Without their encouragement and support, I could not have continued working during my cancer treatment.

One of my dearest friends, Kay Hopkins, has been a close friend and prayer warrior. She encouraged me to write my story and share God's goodness with others.

I cannot forget a good friend, James Shoemake, a member of our Sunday School class. He has been a constant encourager and has urged me to complete the work God began in my spirit.

In addition to the supporters who have prayed and encouraged this endeavor, I remember my pastor, Dr. Steve Rose. I appreciate the visits when I was hospitalized. My church family at First Assembly of God in Muskogee, Oklahoma really stood in the gap for my recovery.

Last but not least, I am thankful for my family members who were so wonderful during my illness and visited me uplifting me with words of encouragement.

My sister, Jerry Bergmann, was a constant source of help and encouragement. She stayed with me for almost a month when I was hospitalized in St. Louis University Hospital in St. Louis, Missouri. I appreciate her so very much. Also, my sister-in-law, Bonnie and my mother-in-law Thelma Rose, were sharing their faith and prayers as well as my brother-in-law, Dewan Rose and his son Mark. I will probably forget some names, but I pray God will bless each person who expressed love and support during these difficult times.

I also want to remember my grandchildren, Tristian, Chelsea, Jacob, and Jonah. It is my deepest desire that the miracles of God's goodness and mercy in my life will impact their lives and cause them to want to be a witness for Jesus Christ all the days of their lives.

Matthew 25:40 tells us "The King will reply whatever you did for one of these brothers of mine, you did for me." Thank you, each and every one of you for your gifts of love.

INTRODUCTION

I AM WRITING my experience with the expectation that it will serve to strengthen and encourage others who are struggling physically and emotionally with similar illnesses. We all suffer illnesses at sometime or another and need the supernatural strength that only comes from God Almighty. Whatever difficulties, be it physical, spiritual or other, God is ready, willing and able to be that miraculous power you need.

Looking back over my life, I realize there were a number of times satan tried to steal my life, but GOD kept me alive to fulfill HIS Purpose. I know, beyond a shadow of doubt, my life belongs to my creator.

God spoke to my heart about three years ago concerning writing a book about the miracles He has performed in my life. Since that time, there have been many circumstances to try and put a stop to this work of faith. The enemy does not want a single person to receive help and strength from this true and simple truth revealed in God's Word. However, with God's help, I have endeavored to share my continuing work of grace with you, the reader of this book.

It is my sincere desire that God will open your spiritual eyes to the wonderful treasures that belong to the children of God. Many times we accept the leftovers or crumbs from The Master's table when it is His desire that we have the choice food, Heaven's best. Most important, please remember that God is not a respecter of persons. What He did for me, He can do the same for you. My prayers go with you as you read my story and the wonderful peace and blessings of being sheltered in His arms.

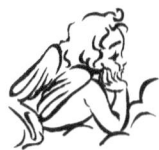

CHAPTER ONE

In The Beginning

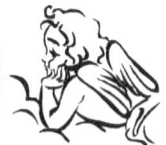

*O*NE OF MY earliest memories of God's healing power is when I was approximately nine years of age. A neighbor's dog bit me on the leg which caused a severe blood infection. I recall having to be absent from school a number of weeks and being unable to wear a shoe. After many painful treatments, I was able to return to school.

At age thirteen, I contracted Scarlet Fever. That was the time when doctors made house calls. Our family physician visited our home every day for two weeks and administered injections of penicillin. Since my parents did not carry health insurance, I was not hospitalized for treatment.

My first encounter with an angel of GOD occurred during this time of being seriously ill with Scarlet Fever. I will always remember waking up and being aware of a comforting presence and hearing my name being called softly several times. It was as if GOD was confirming that HE would always be with me no matter the circumstance.

One special night I recall being very restless with a high fever. I heard a soft voice calling my name and sat straight up in the bed. After seeing I was alone in the room, I called out until my mother came to my bedside. After assuring me she had not called out to me, I realized it had to be an angel of God giving me comfort and strength. Following that close encounter, I began to heal and recover.

Although I passed through the valley of the shadow of death many times, nothing could take me out of GOD'S hands. Romans 8:38 tells us "Nothing can separate us from the love of GOD that is in CHRIST JESUS Our Lord."

I gave my heart to GOD when I was only five years of age. I believe that the enemy of my soul tried many times to steal my life pre-maturely. He knew that, as long as I lived, I would be a witness for GOD.

John 10:10 says "the thief cometh not but to steal, kill and destroy. I have come that they might have life, and have that life more abundantly."

2 Peter 1:3 says "His divine power has given us everything we need for life and godliness through our knowledge of Him who called us by His own glory and goodness. Through these, He has given us His very great and precious promises, so that through them you may participate in the divine nature and escape the corruption in the world caused by evil desires."

I now take you back to the time my third child was born on August 12, 1986. My daughter, Rhonda, was in a breech position. Since I had been in labor for many hours and failed to dilate adequately, the doctor performed a C-section. After my baby was delivered, I began to hemorrhage profusely. I later learned the surgical team had been quite concerned that I might not survive. I knew that God was keeping watch over me once again. He still had unfinished business for me to accomplish.

CHAPTER TWO

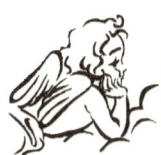 A Sentence Of Death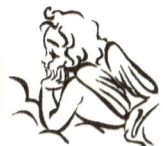

I CAN STILL vividly remember that day in the doctor's office when he pronounced the finding of a malignant tumor in my left breast. The lump had been found during a previous routine mammogram. From that moment until I walked out of the office, it was like watching a drama on television. This could not be happening to me. It had to be a bad dream and I longed to awake. I remember the surgeon telling me the options available to me. I was told to think about it and let him know my decision in a few days.

When my husband and I reached our car, hot tears began to flow down from my eyes as I realized that I was facing one of the most difficult times of my life.

With numerous questions going through my mind, I called out to God "Why is this happening to me? I am one of your children. I try to witness to others. I do my best to live for you. So, why have I received this sentence of death?"

In my weakness, God was strong. The Comforter, The Holy Spirit, began to bring wonderful, comforting words of Bible scriptures to my remembrance. One was I Peter 4:12, "Beloved, think it not strange concerning the fiery trial which is to try you as though some strange thing happened to you, but rejoice inasmuch as you are partakers of Christ's sufferings, that when his glory shall be revealed, you may be glad with exceeding joy."

Another favorite comforting Bible scripture was I Peter 2:21-24. "For even hereunto were you called; because Christ also suffered for us leaving us an example that you should follow his steps, who did no sin, neither was guile found in His mouth. Who His own self bore our sins in His own body on the tree, that we, being dead to sins, should live with righteousness; by whose stripes you were healed." What wonderful words of life!

Through GOD'S holy word, I received supernatural strength and courage to face my enemy of Cancer, Each day I would awake and thank God for my salvation and my healing that He purchased on the cross of Calvary.

I wish I could tell you that God instantly healed my body, though this had been the case in other illnesses. This time, however, God healed my disease through the help of doctors and medicine. I am so thankful for the knowledge and improvements in the treatment of cancer and other diseases. God has indeed blessed our generation with awesome medical technology. The difference in results, however, lies not in men's knowledge, but in the wisdom of God.

In the days that followed, I did a lot of research on breast cancer. I searched the internet for information and talked to other women who had gone through breast surgeries and cancer treatments. My family tried their best to encourage me and help me through these dark days.

After much prayer and research, I finally made the decision to undergo lumpectomy surgery to be followed by chemotherapy and radiation. My surgeon had told me that lumpectomy surgeries had proved to be as successful as a total mastectomy in several statistics. So, I had elected to undergo the least radical intervention.

The oncology doctors recommended that I receive chemotherapy to be followed by radiation. I had known people who had little difficulty during chemotherapy. However, treatment proved to be a little different in my situation. There were days I actually felt as if my very life was being drained from my body. During the days immediately following treatments, I literally had to force down every bite of food, but I knew it was necessary in order to keep up my strength.

Whenever you struggle with a life threatening disease or injury, you really learn to appreciate the little things you once took for granted. Every day becomes a celebration of life. You wake up in the mornings saying, "Thank God for another day," instead of "Oh God, another day."

CHAPTER THREE

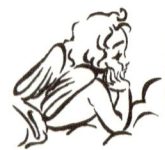

Only Believe

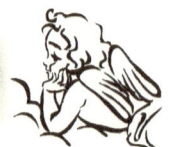

ON'T BE DISCOURAGED if you don't see the manifestation of your complete healing. I believed God had begun a work of healing in my body and would be faithful to complete it in His time. Jesus himself said in Matthew 21:21, "If you have faith and doubt not, you shall say to this mountain, be thou removed and cast into the sea, it shall be done."

Thank GOD for an employer who allowed me to work at home during my chemotherapy treatments. I forced my tired, aching body to get out of bed each day, and with God's help, I managed to work at least 30 hours per week following my treatments. Following a few days at home, I would return to the office and work duties.

I really empathize with anyone who is forced to endure chemo. Because the strong medicines destroy good blood cells as well as cancer cells, the treatments leave the body in an extremely weakened condition. I remember feeling so weak at times, I could barely walk or think.

On one particular occasion, I drove to my office planning to try and work, only to discover I was too weak to even sit at my desk. A dear friend and co-worker ended up having to drive me back to my home. Following that incident, my oncologist administered injections to help rebuild my immune system.

The normal routine for my chemotherapy treatments began. One day I would receive the chemotherapy medicines, and the following day would be the time when I received medicines to rebuild my blood cells. Had it not been for my excellent insurance coverage, my family could not have afforded the expensive cost of the required injections. I now understand the extreme importance of adequate medical coverage. If you are one of the people needing cancer treatment and do not have required insurance coverage, please know there are organizations to help pay for the necessary drugs you need for treatment.

Yes, these were difficult days. However, I kept my mind on healing and being "cancer free". I cannot speak for others, but I definitely believe continuing to work at my job helped in my recovery. Working kept my mind busy and not dwelling on how weak and sick I actually felt. Also, the fellowship with my co-workers was also very encouraging. I knew they were pulling with me in my battle to survive.

I gained a new appreciation for the hair covering my head. As long as I could remember, one thing I had been blessed with was a thick, curly head of dark hair. A couple of weeks after my first chemo treatment, my hair started turning loose in handfuls. Every morning my pillow was covered with strands of hair. I had never considered myself as a vain person, but looking at my thinning strands of hair was a hard knock to my femininity. One morning I asked my husband, Bob, to shave my head. After looking at my bald head in the mirror, tears began to flood my eyes. The face looking back at me seemed like a stranger. I felt like part of my being was now missing.

Thank GOD for wigs! I soon became very familiar with my new head of hair, but when I was at home, I chose to go natural. My wonderful husband tried to make me feel good by telling me I still looked beautiful to him. Had it not been for the love and support of my husband and family, I could not have made it some days. I can still remember my husband holding my hand at bedtime and praying for my strength and healing. He told me many times he wished he could take my place.

A most unusual thing occurred shortly after my recovery from the breast cancer. My husband, Bob, was diagnosed with carcinoma in his left breast. It was decided that a total mastectomy would be performed in his case. My husband's surgery was a complete success, and he did not need to receive any chemotherapy or radiation treatment. I teased him a few times and told him he was just having sympathy for my cancer ordeal.

Following his surgery and my treatment, we both became "cancer survivors."

Following my last chemo treatment, my family helped me celebrate a huge milestone in my recovery.

It was one of the greatest victories I have ever won. I know I could not have endured without God's never changing love and strength. Hebrews 4:15 says, "For we do not have a high priest who is unable to sympathize with our weaknesses, but we have one who has been tempted in every way, just as we are, yet without sin. Let us then approach the throne of grace with confidence, so that we may receive mercy and find grace to help in our time of need."

When I fought my battle with breast cancer in 2002, I thought that would be the worst battle I would ever have to fight in my life. After six months of chemo therapy and radiation following breast surgery, I learned that God was my constant supply of strength and healing. I continued working at my job as a benefits analyst in health insurance through the cancer treatments and had really learned to appreciate each day of life. All my health physicals were good.

Immediately after completing the last chemo treatment I was sent to the hospital to make sure the treatment had eradicated the cancer. After many mammograms, I was finally told by the technicians they were not sure the tumor was completely gone because they had found another lump in my breast. We were about to leave the hospital when they advised me that I needed to go to the radiology building where they could obtain a clearer image. At this point, I was on the verge of tears and my tender breast felt as though it had been smashed by an iron door. I began praying earnestly for another miracle as I repeated Bible scriptures in my mind.

My husband had driven me to the radiological center for the tests, and he had to leave to pick up our daughter from school. The radiologist had taken a few more images which were being examined to obtain the final results. In what seemed like an eternity, the technician was finally able to tell me all that was visible on the mammograms was only scar tissue. Praise God.

I wondered many times if there might have been traces of the malignant growth when the first images were examined.

Whatever the case, God had completely vanished the disease from my body.

When my husband arrived to pick me up at the center, I was smiling and elated to tell him and my daughter the wonderful news of my healing. My family helped me celebrate another milestone in my complete recovery from cancer. I know I could not have endured without God's never changing love and strength. Hebrews 4:15 says, "For we do not have a high priest who is unable to sympathize with our weaknesses, but we have one who has been tempted in every way, just as we are, yet without sin."

Next came radiation therapy. This was performed five days per week, Mondays through Fridays, for six weeks. I was able to keep working at my job without the severe side effects I had endured while taking chemotherapy treatments.

After completing the final radiation treatment, my family and I rejoiced together. After numerous testing, it was finally announced that my body was now "cancer free". I was so elated that I began to dance for joy. I finally began to feel "normal" once again. If you have been through a similar illness, you can identify with these feelings. There just are not adequate words to express the joy and relief you feel. I praised my God for His everlasting mercy and grace.

If you currently, or in the future, receive a diagnosis of cancer or another life threatening illness, do not despair. The God who created us also knows how to heal us. I encourage you to read all the healing scriptures in The Bible and also read books written by people like myself who have experienced similar illnesses and are now living testimonies of the greatness of God's love.

I wish I could tell you that "I lived happily ever after", but that will not happen until I reach my eternal, heavenly home. Meanwhile, each one of us must run this race of life.

After you have been diagnosed with a life threatening disease such as cancer, it becomes easy to be plagued by fears of that disease returning. Many times satan tried to bring doubts to my mind. Every time I encountered pain or sickness, the enemy would torment my mind with thoughts in an attempt to destroy my faith.

During these times that tried my faith, I came against my enemy with God's word. Jesus left us the supreme example when he was tempted by satan in the desert following fasting and praying. Matthew 4:2-10 tells how Jesus used God's word to answer the devil. Then verse 11 tells us the devil left him.

While Jesus lived on the earth, He was in human form and was subject to the same limitations of the flesh like you and me. Therefore, if Jesus used the Holy Scriptures to conquer the enemy, You and I need to follow His example and tell the enemy "It is written".

I cannot count the number of times the Holy Spirit of God brought comforting scriptures to my remembrance. God's promises are as real today as they were when Jesus walked the earth more than two thousand years ago and performed many miracles. The Bible tells us in Hebrews 13:8, "Jesus Christ is the same yesterday, today and forever".

Philippians 4:6 tells us "Do not be anxious about anything, but in everything, by prayer and petition, with thanksgiving present your requests to God." Matthew 21:22 tells us "If you believe, you will receive whatever you ask in prayer."

There is a vast supply of God's promises to us. Every time a negative thought comes to my mind, I think about a Bible verse to counteract the doubt and fear. I say the verse aloud. I tell the enemy that I refuse to accept any idea that is not in line with God's word. I even go so far as to tell satan he is a liar just like he was in the Garden of Eden. Then, I say "I know I am healed because God's Word says I am, and God cannot lie."

CHAPTER FOUR

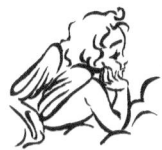

Miracle Baby

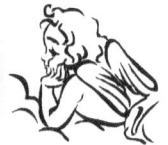

*I*N THE EARLY part of 2008, our youngest daughter, Rhonda, and her husband Bradley, were expecting a baby. The early testing had revealed a problem, so she had been sent to a specialist.

I will never forget the look of despair on my daughter's face when she was told her baby had gastroschisis, a condition where the baby's intestines are outside the body. The doctor explained to Rhonda that she had delivered a number of babies with this birth defect that survived to live healthy lives. It was further explained that her pregnancy would be monitored closely to ensure the baby was growing and developing properly. As soon as the baby was born, it would be necessary to perform surgery to place the intestines back inside the body. The baby would need to be in I C U for 14-16 weeks until his system was functioning normally and that it would take at least two surgeries to return the intestines in their proper place.

It was an enormous load to carry. As soon as we walked out of the doctor's office my daughter started to cry. Her father, husband and I all assured her the baby would be alright.

God spoke to my heart to buy an outfit for the baby in order to show that we believed God would work a miracle for this special little boy. There were some difficult moments during our daughter's pregnancy. But God helped this "little miracle" to develop into a precious baby boy.

I will never forget my first glimpse of our newborn infant grandson. He was enclosed in a large incubator with a covering over his stomach. It was a very emotional time for our whole family. We had to trust in our spiritual sight, not our natural sight.

During the time Jacob was hospitalized in N.I.C.U., my daughter, Rhonda and her husband, Bradley, drove to the hospital every day to spend time with their baby boy. This was very difficult for them since the hospital was 60 miles away from their home town.

However, they were determined to spend as much time as possible with their newborn son. I believe this effort of love helped our grandson to heal and recover quicker than the doctors had anticipated. Our home church, as well as other churches, had been praying for our daughter and our unborn grandson for many months. After Jacob's birth, prayers continued to be offered in his behalf.

My husband and I, as well as my son-in-law's family, visited Jacob in the N.I.C.U. as often as possible. The first time we visited following the surgery was really heartbreaking to see our tiny grandson encircled in a maze of tubes and wires. It was all I could do to keep the tears from overflowing my eyes. I will always remember the first time I got to hold our newborn grandson and feed him a bottle. All I could do was whisper words of love and thanksgiving to God for his miracle of life. Psalms 37:4 says, "Delight yourself in the Lord, and He will give you the desires of your heart." What a wonderful promise!

After Jacob was delivered, he was rushed into surgery to correct the problem with the intestines. The doctors were amazed at how quickly he recovered. He was able to be released from the hospital after only two weeks. It was necessary to perform only one additional surgery a few months later to repair a hernia.

GOD'S goodness still is evident today in our grandson, Jacob's, life. He is a normal, active and healthy little four-year-old boy. With the exception of his missing belly button, he is just like all little boys his age. We continue to praise God for our little miracle.

Two years later, our family was blessed with another grandson. This baby was born without any complications, praise God! Little Jonah has been a sweet bundle of joy and blessing from God. We continue to thank God daily for His bountiful supply and trust God that He will hold our children and grandchildren in the shelter of His arms. We believe God's Word that says, "Train up a child in the way he should go, and when he is old, he will not depart from it." This is found in Proverbs 22:6.

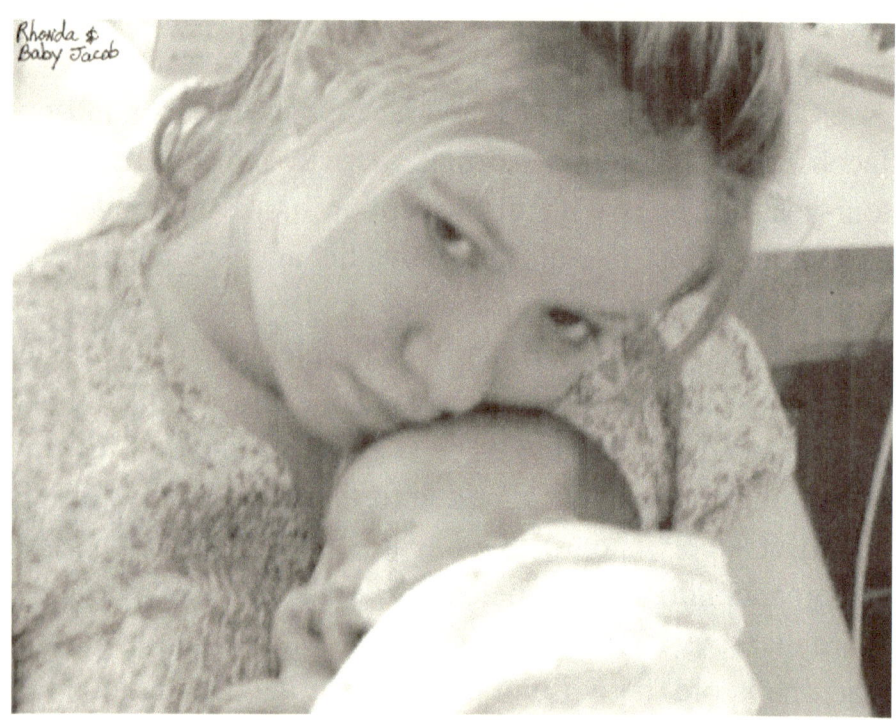

Rhonda &
Baby Jacob

CHAPTER FIVE

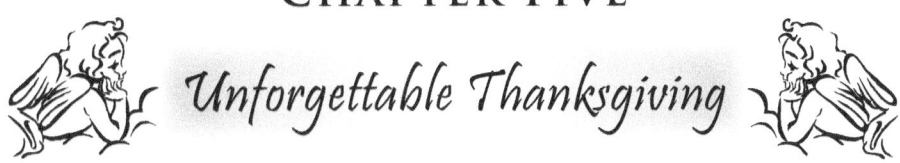

Unforgettable Thanksgiving

NOW IT WAS two days before Thanksgiving the same year, 2008. Our church had its regular Wednesday night service on Tuesday night since a lot of the people would be preparing for Thanksgiving.

I went to bed Tuesday night thinking about how much God had blessed our family. Approximately 3:00AM Wednesday morning, I awoke with the worst headache I had ever experienced, and I found I was unable to move my neck. There was the most intense pain and pressure in the base of my skull. The pain was unbearable. I woke my husband and we rushed to the emergency room at the hospital.

If you have ever visited an emergency room department, you are aware that a patient will not receive any medications for pain until they have been examined by the attending physician. It seemed like an eternity before a doctor finally arrived to evaluate my pain. During this time period, I was vomiting, and the pain was excruciating.

The doctor on duty said it was probably a pinched nerve and would give me a shot for pain and prescribe pain medication, and it would probably go away and I could go home. I didn't accept that diagnosis and told the doctor there was something terribly wrong with my neck, and I wanted it x-rayed. This really surprised the doctor, but at insistence, I had an x-ray of my neck done. After reading the x-ray, he came back out and said there was something definitely wrong and would do a cat-scan. The next thing I knew I was being life flighted to a larger hospital in Tulsa, Oklahoma. The neurologist performed an arteriogram along with another MRI, and determined that I had a brain aneurysm in the stem at the base of my brain. The neurosurgeon felt uncomfortable operating on the aneurysm but knew of a neurosurgeon that had done this type of surgery before. The next morning, which was Thanksgiving, I was life flighted to St. Louis, Mo. I thought I would go into surgery as soon as I got there. However, I soon learned that was not going to happen for another ten days. I was placed in a private room with no lighting or television or any kind of sound during this time and was also kept under sedation because of the seriousness of the situation. The doctor explained that this was necessary because the blood clot had to resolve itself before any kind of operation could be done. The location of the aneurysm also made it very difficult to operate. Since I couldn't do anything, this was a great time for me to pray, and I prayed a lot. It may sound unreal, but I really wasn't fearful. I knew God was with me and that he was taking care of me.

My oldest daughter, Candee, flew in from Texas to be with me a few days and my sister stayed until a few days before Christmas. My husband was with me the whole time. The rest of my family and friends were unable to visit me during this time, and I sure missed them, especially at Christmas. I was so sick, I hardly knew when Christmas came and went, and this is my favorite time of the year. Also, during this time, my husband kept in touch with the pastor and the men's group at our home church.

CHAPTER SIX

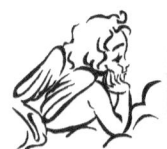

Life Or Death

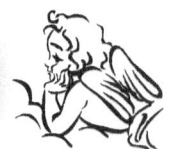

*B*ACK TO THE surgery. The surgeon told my husband the surgery would last approximately 8 hours. It lasted 12 hours. The surgeon explained to my husband that the aneurysm was larger than they expected, and they had to put two clamps on it. I found out later, after the surgery was completed that the doctor told my husband prior to the surgery that I may not make it, and if I did, I may be in a vegetative state the rest of my life or be paralyzed. My husband told the surgeon that he would be praying and that God would bring me through in good shape.

I remember waking up after the surgery and hearing a nurse saying "She has angels all around her." I was blessed with wonderful, caring nurses while I was in I.C.U. I felt God's presence hovering over me. It was a very difficult time as well. Because of all the strong drugs given to keep me sedated, I suffered through horrible hallucinations and bad dreams. Sometimes it was difficult to know what was real and what wasn't.

One night I awoke to a voice asking me if I knew where I was. Through the bright lights and everyone dressed in white,

I replied "Is this Heaven?" The nurse laughed and said "No honey, this is the hospital."

It seemed, at times, like I was in a different world. There were nurses that had the appearance of people I worked with in the office. To this day, they seemed very real. My life in the hospital seemed to be sleeping, pain, I.V.s, needles, Cat Scans, and people always asking me if I knew my name and where I was.

Imagine waking up with your eyes swollen shut, a big contraption around your head, a breathing tube down your throat, and your hands in restraints. I could hear my husband's voice telling me that he loved me, and that I had made it through the surgery alright.

If you have ever been through surgery, you can identify with my feelings of just wanting to return to sleep. At that point, you just want to make the pain vanish and return to that peaceful, dream like state. During the course of the next several hours, I would awake to voices asking me if I knew where I was. I would try to answer, but the tube down my throat made it impossible to talk. I wondered why someone did not take the device out of my throat. I just wanted the foreign device removed.

After three or four days had passed, I was finally relieved of the irritating ventilator. My throat was sore and scratchy, but it was a wonderful relief to be able to breathe normally again. My lips had become cracked and swollen, and I longed for a cool drink of water; however, this was not to be a reality.

It soon became apparent there was a problem with my swallowing. Every time I tried to swallow a sip of water or eat a bit of ice, I would begin choking. After several days without nourishment, other than the intravenous fluids, I began to get very hungry. The thoughts of my favorite foods began to torment my empty stomach. My mouth felt as if I had been walking through the dry, parched desert in search of coveted water.

It was finally decided that a temporary feeding tube would be inserted through my nose running down into my throat. Several attempts were required before the device worked properly. The device caused me to feel extremely nauseous. It was necessary, however, if my starving body was to receive necessary nourishment. This was a short term solution to the problem.

During the days following my lengthy surgery, it was determined that I also had damage to muscles and nerves controlling my voice. I could not understand why everyone had difficulty hearing me when I spoke to them. The damage had occurred during the surgery to repair the aneurysm. It was decided that another surgery would be necessary to try and repair my voice volume.

In order to repair this damage, I was advised that a wedge would be inserted in my throat.

For this second surgery, I was given conscious sedation. At different times the surgical team would get me to talk in order to determine the volume of my voice. I was monitored very closely for several days, and it appeared that this procedure had helped my voice problem.

During the post surgical time period, I discovered that I also had a hearing loss. It sounded like my ears were filled with water. It felt similar to being in a deep well. It was suggested that I follow up with an E.N.T. specialist when I returned home. I remember thinking, "It just gets better all the time."

Everyone kept telling me how blessed I was to be alive, but to be truthful, I had mixed feelings about the whole situation. I will elaborate more on this subject a little bit later.

I took one step forward and another step back. The volume of my voice improved, but my swallowing muscles were still not working properly. Every swallow study revealed I was still aspirating into my lungs, which can lead to pneumonia. At this point, it was suggested that a feeding tube be placed into my stomach. At first, I rebelled at the idea of a feeding tube, but I was growing weary of being in the hospital. It had now been four weeks, and I longed to return home and sleep in my own bed once again.

After reluctantly agreeing to another surgery, I decided this was necessary in order to regain my strength and independence. After the placement of the feeding tube, I began to receive my nourishment via a tube in my stomach. At least, I was closer to getting released from the hospital to return home.

Before being released from the hospital in St. Louis, I was to be transported to rehab in my home town to strengthen my weakened body and help with my swallowing therapy. Each day seemed to drag by endlessly. I began to cry and beg to return home.

Arrangements were finally in place for me to be transferred by ambulance to our home town hospital in Muskogee,

Oklahoma, where I was to receive rehabilitation. St. Louis University Hospital had been my home away from home for five weeks, and Christmas had passed by without the warmth spent with family and friends.

CHAPTER SEVEN

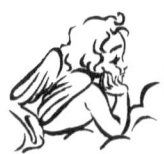 *The Long Ride Home*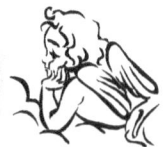

*I*T WAS DECEMBER 31, 2008, the last day of the year. I would soon be homeward bound. Hallelujah!

The long ambulance ride proved to be very stressful for me. Before the ambulance had arrived at the hospital, I was nauseated and vomiting. The hospital staff had assured me I would be given something to help out on the long journey to my home town of Muskogee, Oklahoma. Soon after being prepared for my ambulance trip, I asked for some medication to help combat the nausea I had been experiencing. I was told that they did not carry any medications in the ambulance. When the back of your skull has a large incision, you feel every bump in the road. Between the pain in my head and the nausea in my stomach, it felt as if there was a conspiracy to make this trip one of torment.

At long last, the ambulance arrived at our final destination. I don't think I was ever so happy to learn I was back in my home town. I had done a lot of praying on the trip home, and God was faithful to see us safe and sound. That last day, December 31, 2008, ended on a joyful note after a very trying time period that had begun the day before Thanksgiving.

That evening I had a wonderful visit from my pastor, Dr. Steve Rose, the pastor of Muskogee First Assembly, as well as my family and friends. Tears of joy ran down my face as we had a sweet reunion with one another. Thank you God for your keeping power and your everlasting grace and mercy. I had a new appreciation for the little things that we all take for granted.

The first day of 2009 was a challenge for me. After so many weeks of lying in a hospital bed, my body was in a very weakened condition. It was time to force my inactive muscles to become strong and active once again.

One of the side effects of my damaged swallowing muscles was the production of excessive amounts of mucous. I was constantly having to suction out mucous, or I tried to cough up the choking secretions.

In addition to the irritation caused by the excessive secretions, this condition also caused me to be nauseated and caused vomiting. It sometimes seemed like a never ending cycle.

After a week of rehabilitation and trying to force my weakened body to perform normal, routine activities, I was finally released from the rehab center at the hospital to return home.

CHAPTER EIGHT

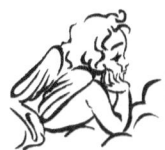 *Home Sweet Home!*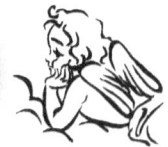

NOTHING WAS SO great as coming home. I had lost over twenty pounds during my stay at St Louis University Hospital and was very weak from the ordeal. I could barely walk, but I was so thankful. I knew God had kept me alive for some reason.

I learned there had been countless people praying for me during this period. I know that it was all those prayers that kept me here. I will be forever thankful for my church that prayed for me. My husband told me later that he was in constant touch with my pastor keeping him up to date on my progress.

I have been told many times by my friends and doctors that I am a walking miracle. However, when I first came home from the hospital, I didn't much feel like a miracle. I talked funny, I couldn't eat or drink anything, I had to be fed through a feeding tube installed in my stomach, and my hearing was affected. I remember asking God "Why did you leave me here like this? Why did this have to happen? I know you could have prevented this from happening. How is this going to work for my good?" I had a lot of doubt and questions. I still don't have all the answers, but I know God loves me and has been with me through everything, and I know this is going to work for my good.

The next few days was spent trying to get my strength back and doing simple things like walking and bathing. The thing that bothered me most, was not being able to eat or drink anything. My mouth was extremely dry and my lips were cracked and chapped from lack of not being able to drink. I watched my family eating, and the aroma from the food really made me hungry. I had to be satisfied with liquid nourishment through the feeding tube.

I was sick at my stomach a lot the first few weeks after returning home. The constant large amounts of swallowing mucous only added to my misery.

On top of everything, I could barely hear anything and my speech had been affected as well. I was constantly coughing up mucous. I kept wondering why God had allowed me to live in such a miserable state of being.

I know from experience that it is really easy to fall into a deep pit of self pity. Whenever I was having these feelings, I discovered the best answer to this problem was to read God's promises and look ahead to the end result. In other words, we need to live by faith and not what we currently see or feel. This is one of the most difficult truths for we as humans to grasp. Since we tend to be controlled by our natural senses, it is a new experience to operate by spiritual truths.

Don't ever lose your goal of being healed. If you hold fast to your faith in God, He will see you through whatever trial you may encounter. I have learned to keep my eyes fixed on the answer and not the question. God never promised life would be easy, but He did promise to never leave us nor forsake us.

Since GOD had already helped me through other illnesses and difficulties, I was more confident that He would see me through this crisis as well. Each time we exercise our spiritual muscles by believing God's Word, we become stronger, much like lifting weights. We start out small and work up to heavier weights. The more we work our spiritual muscles, the stronger they become.

I was having a really good pity party shortly after my return home. Instead of counting my blessings, I was focusing on the problems. After a difficult morning of being nauseated and choking on excessive mucous, I blurted out, "Why did God leave me here like this? I can't talk right, I can't eat or drink anything, and I can barely hear." My husband, Bob, immediately rebuked my complaints. He said, "I never want to hear you talk like that again. The doctors say that you are a walking miracle." I asked God to forgive me through hot tears of sorrow. I ask my Heavenly Father to forgive me and help me focus on my blessings. I am so thankful my God understands and forgives. He knows we are but flesh, and He is touched with the feelings of our infirmities. This is found in Hebrews 4:15.

CHAPTER NINE

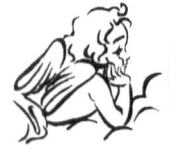 *A Very Grateful Lady*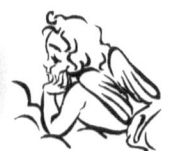

I WILL BE eternally grateful for friends and church brothers and sisters who showered me and my family with their acts of love. Delicious meals were prepared and brought to our home, but I was tormented by the alluring aromas of home cooked foods that I was unable to eat. At this time, the feeding tube was my only source of nourishment, and my mouth watered for a taste of real food.

While in the hospital, I lost over twenty pounds. Most of my clothes hung on my slender frame like a tent. The frail, skinny person staring back at me in the mirror only added sadness to my already grieving spirit. The doctors at the rehab facility prescribed home health to help strengthen my weakened body. I began a regimen of exercises for my physical body as well as speech therapy for my damaged throat muscles. I had my work cut out for me, but I was determined to conquer this giant with God's help. Following three to four weeks of home health assistance, I began to gain some strength, and my voice began to gain some volume as well.

I began to perform light housework and started preparing meals for my family. This was the most difficult job for me since I was unable to eat or drink any foods at that time. The aromas of cooking foods tormented my taste buds. I had to watch my family as they enjoyed eating the dishes that I could only dream of savoring.

As the time passed, my speech therapist advised me to start sipping small amounts of liquids. The small sips of liquid were like drinking from an oasis in the desert. I began to drink small sips each day. Next came small bites of food such as pudding which were easy to swallow. These soft foods seemed to slide down my throat easily. At this point, the speech therapist suggested I be evaluated by means of a swallow study which would be performed on an out patient basis.

The day of the swallowing test arrived. During this procedure, I was required to drink some small amounts of thickened liquid and also to swallow small amounts of different foods. Whenever I swallowed, it was projected on a screen. To my disappointment, I was told the swallow study had revealed that I was still aspirating into my lungs. It was therefore recommended I keep the feeding tube for nourishment. I was more determined to rid myself of "the tube". Each day I faithfully performed the exercises to strengthen my throat muscles. One of the daily, routine drills was to stick out my tongue all the way and swallow as hard as possible. Try it. It is not as easy as you would think. I was encouraged to do this at least one hundred times daily. I found this almost impossible to do in the beginning; however, after many attempts, I was finally able to achieve the desired results. I remembered the scripture, "I can do all things through Christ who strengthens me." Philippians 4:13.

CHAPTER TEN

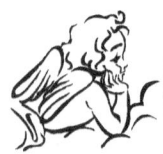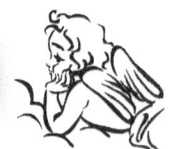

A Visit From God

*T*HE FIRST MONTH after I arrived home was a mixture of sweet and bitterness. I slept a lot, cried a lot and prayed a lot. I believed in healing and I constantly prayed that God would heal me. I longed to be able to eat and drink like "normal people". I hardly ever talked on the phone due to my hearing problem. I kept in touch with my family and friends via the e-mail. One morning after waking to the beginning of another miserable day, I prayed as sincerely as I knew how. I said "Jesus, I know you can heal me. Whatever is keeping me from being healed, please show me." As I prayed that prayer, the Holy Spirit showed up. As plain as if Jesus were there in my room with me. He said "Remember I have already purchased your salvation and healing on the cross. YOU HAVE ALREADY BEEN HEALED, SO ACT LIKE IT." At that instant, faith rose up in me. I repeated "By your stripes I have been healed".

The Holy Spirit reminded me how Peter's mother-in-law had been sick with a fever. When she was prayed for, she arose from her sick bed and ministered to those of her house. Prompted by the Holy Spirit, I got out of bed and cooked breakfast for my husband. The food smelled so good. God spoke to me as plain as if He were in person. He said to me "What would you do if you were healed?" I replied "I would eat breakfast". Once again He said, "you are healed. Now act like it." That was the beginning of another miracle. I cooked a soft egg and ate some crispy bacon. I took small bites and chewed thoroughly. I drank a few sips of tea. That simple breakfast was like manna from heaven to my mouth. After that step of faith, I began to eat other foods.

The doctors told me that I was at high risk for pneumonia because of the swallowing difficulties. I was told I would probably have to use the feeding tube for another year. But my faith in God gave me strength and hope that He would keep me in good health.

Since my eating and drinking liquids got progressively better, I requested to have the feeding tube removed. After a swallow study was completed at the hospital, I was told that I was aspirating into my lungs, and it was too dangerous to have the feeding tube removed. I was disappointed, but my faith was assuring me that God would continue to strengthen my swallowing muscles. However, by faith and listening to the Holy Spirit, I had already been eating solid foods a few weeks prior. I'm not saying that everyone should do this. You should listen to the Holy Spirit and follow his instructions.

Through the weeks that followed, God gave me many scriptures that would strengthen my faith in His healing and purpose for my life. My favorite Bible scripture is the 91st Psalm from where I received the title of this book. I read this chapter over and over. These precious promises became my confession and shelter. This chapter had also been a great source of strength during my breast cancer diagnosis and treatment some seven years earlier. I also read other bible scriptures on healing such as Mark 11:23-24 "If anyone says to this mountain, Go and throw yourself into the sea" and does not doubt in his heart but believes what he says, it will be done for him." 'Therefore I tell you, whatever you ask for in prayer, believe that you have received it and it will be yours.'" Also in Matthew 8:14-17. It says "When Jesus came into Peter's house, He saw Peter's mother lying in bed with a fever. He touched her hand and the fever left her and she got up and began to wait on them. When evening came, many who were demon possessed were brought to Him and He drove out the spirit with a word and healed the sick."

Along with GOD'S word I also read several books written about healing. Even though I didn't see the manifestation of my total healing, I would wake up each morning and thank God for his healing and salvation in my life. I believed that God's word was true, even if I didn't see my total healing and deliverance. That's what faith is . . . . Acting like you're healed because God's word says you are.

In May of 2009, after I had returned home from the hospital in January, my E. N. T. doctor said he thought it would be safe to remove my feeding tube. That was exciting, and what a relief to be free of "the tube".

Every time I have an appointment with one of the physicians, they always say that I am a walking miracle.

I don't have all the answers, and I'm not sure why this happened, or why God left me here instead of taking me to be with Him. All I know, is that my life is not my own, and for some purpose, God wanted me here to tell other people going through similar experiences, that Jesus paid the price for our salvation and healing. We don't have to live in sin or diseases and sickness. He purchased all that we need on Calvary's rugged cross. I am nobody special, just a woman who believed God's word. I have truly been sheltered in the arms of Almighty God.

Bible scripture JOHN 16:33 Jesus said "In this world you will have trouble. But take heart! I overcame the world". James 5:14-16 tells us "Is anyone of you sick? He should call the elders of the church to pray over him and anoint him with oil in the name of the Lord. And the prayer offered in faith will make the sick person well, the Lord will raise him up. If he has sinned, he will be forgiven."

CHAPTER ELEVEN

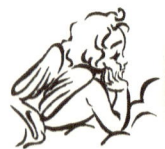
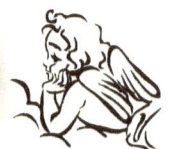

Angel Rescue

*H*AVE YOU EVER been rescued by an angel? You probably have without realizing it. Just as we, as natural parents, try to protect our children from danger, so our Heavenly Father protects us, His children, as well. Perhaps you will recall a time when you were trying to drive to an appointment or a specific place and were delayed by traffic, or for some other reason, you were late in arriving at your destination. Many times these delays may have kept you from being involved in a serious automobile accident or other catastrophe.

I want to share two different near death encounters with you:

The first close encounter occurred approximately thirty years ago. Our family was taking a vacation trip to Eureka Springs in the Ozark Mountains. A pop-up camper was being pulled behind our car. If you are familiar with this area of the country, you know there are many curves and steep hills along the highway.

One side of the road was solid rock, and the other side was a steep, deep drop-off which went straight down. As we were traveling along this stretch of highway, a huge semi-trailer truck came barreling around the approaching curve onto our side of the road.

There was not sufficient time to think about what to do next. Somehow, my husband managed to get over to the right where there was a narrow ditch. The semi continued to veer in our direction. We were all petrified as the left side of the camper was hit and stripped of all the metal trim and utility connections. As we sat glued to our seats, the semi continued on without even slowing down in speed.

When we finally collected our wits, we had a chance to look around and survey the damages. The car that had been following behind the semi truck stopped to make sure we were not injured. As we all looked around us, we began to see how close we had come to being another traffic fatality.

To this day, my husband is amazed at how quickly he reacted and hit the ditch just in time. This was the only thing that kept us from being a part of the high, rock wall. The camper was the only thing that was damaged. If my husband had moved the other direction, our car would have fallen down the steep embankment. If he had waited a few seconds longer to hit the ditch, the truck would have struck us in a head-on collision.

We had always made it a practice to have prayer before leaving our driveway at home and embarking on a trip. We had prayed for God's protection before we left home, and we were so thankful for the mercies of God's rescue. Even our children, who were young at the time, recognized that God had worked a miracle for all of our family.

Not only had God performed a miracle in our behalf, but the driver of the semi was also rescued. When we saw that huge truck come swinging around the curve, only one side of the truck's wheels were on the road. The other side of the wheels were off the edge of the road containing the steep drop-off. I don't know if the driver ever took notice that he had been part of a supernatural miracle or not, but all who witnessed the incident knew this to be a truth. It is so true to God's Word that the angels of God encamp round about those who fear Him. This is found in Psalms 34:7.

CHAPTER TWELVE

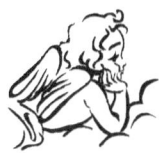 *Another God Encounter*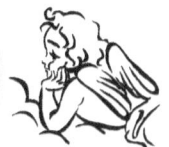

MANY TIMES THROUGHOUT my life I have recognized the super-natural power of God at work. Not only has God healed my body many times, but He has also protected me from many dangers as well.

One special God encounter occurred three years ago. My husband and I had been visiting our daughter, Candee, in Killeen, Texas. After a wonderful time together, we were on our way back home. My husband, Bob, was driving at this time. We were headed north on the inside lane of a four-lane highway. There was a concrete wall on the left side which separated the highway. I happened to look up and notice a semi-trailer truck on our right side. There was a car behind us, and a car was in front of us. As we were driving along, I looked and saw the semi to our right start to veer over into our car. I knew there was nowhere to go, so I closed my eyes and braced for the impact. At this point, I was aware that our car was being moved. It was as if we were suspended in time. As I opened my eyes, to my surprise, our car was ahead of the semi truck, and there was still a car in front of us.

I asked my husband "What just happened?" He replied that he wasn't sure. He, too, remembered seeing the semi start to veer over into our lane. He knew he could not move left due to the concrete wall, so he, too, had prepared for the impact collision with the semi truck. He, like me, was very surprised to see the semi now behind our car and in our lane. We both recognized that this had to be a God encounter. It was as if something had picked up our car and placed it ahead of the semi.

We are still unsure as to what exactly occurred. One thing we knew for sure is that God had rescued us one more time by using His miraculous power.

So, dear reader, do not give up hope or be discouraged. God is still in control of your life. Nothing can take us out of His hands, not even death. He has conquered that foe as well. One scripture telling us this truth is Hosea 13:14.

He has also promised never to leave us, see Deut.31:6. I Cor. 15:54-55 tells us ""Death has been swallowed up in victory. Where O death is your sting?"

EPILOGUE

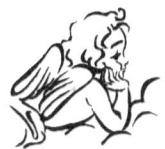

My Purpose

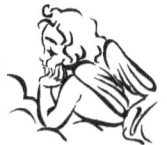

T HE MESSAGE OF my story was birthed by the Holy Spirit. I am just an ordinary person who God is using to bring forth His message of hope and peace to those who are discouraged and depressed and wonder why they are facing an illness, a problem or a seemingly impossible situation in which there is no way out.

As I have said many times before, I don't have all the answers, but God does. Like the title of my book, I love to picture God's arms sheltering me and protecting me from the storms of this life. Every time I start to feel discouraged, I read Psalms 91, my favorite chapter in the Bible.

There are many of God's promises in the Bible. Find the promise that fits your need and stand on that word. When I was unable to eat or drink, I found a scripture in the Bible. I repeated the scripture daily until I was able to eat and drink once again. It will work for you too. Give God a chance.

At last, dear reader, I earnestly hope my story has given you a new determination to walk by faith and not by sight. 2 Corinthians 6:2 tells us that NOW is the time of God's favor and salvation.

Isaiah 53: 4-5 tells us Jesus took up our infirmities and carried our sorrows, He was pierced by our transgressions, He was crushed for our iniquities, the punishment that brought us peace was upon Him, and by his wounds we are healed. Praise be to God! The price for our healing and salvation has already been paid. All you and I have to do is open our hearts and minds to receive God's gift.

I love 2Corinthians 5:1-10. It tells us that if our earthly bodies are destroyed, we have an eternal house in Heaven not built by human hands. When we are at home in our present bodies, we are away from the Lord. So God has given his Spirit as a deposit of what is to come.

As my daughter, Rhonda, and I were reminiscing about the events that occurred almost four years ago, we both cried and shared our hearts as we thanked God for His Thanksgiving miracle.

Thanks to God's healing touch, I have had the joy of attending my oldest daughter, Candee's graduation from nursing school, one granddaughter's graduation from high school, another granddaughter's graduation from college, the birth of my second grandson, and just last month, the wedding of my oldest granddaughter, Tristian.

God's goodness and mercy will follow me all the days of my life, and like David said in his 23rd Psalm, "I will dwell in the house of the Lord forever." You can't top that promise. The best is yet to come.

There is really no end to this story. It is actually just the beginning.

When I accepted Jesus Christ as my Lord and Savior, my name was written in God's Book of Life. He will be with me in this life as well as the eternal life to come. It is a "win win" situation. As a child of God, I can walk in victory from here throughout all eternity.

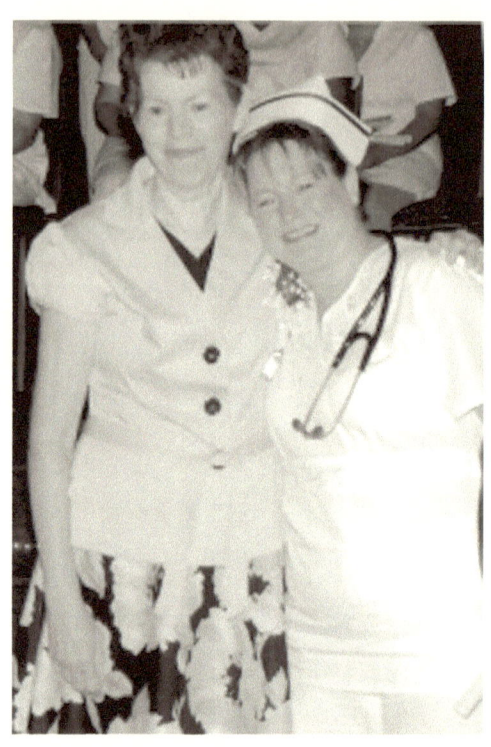

Daughter Candee's graduation from nursing school

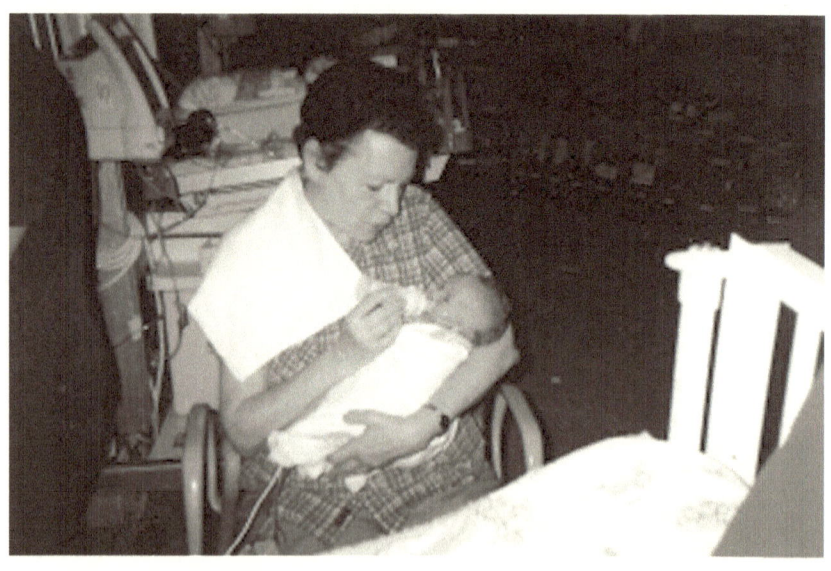

Grandma feeding Jacob in N.I.C.U.

Grandsons

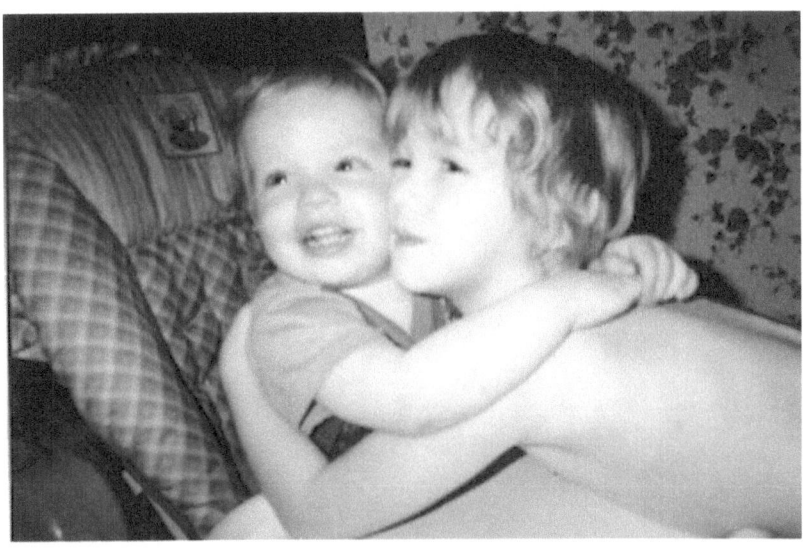

Jacob hugging brother, Jonah.

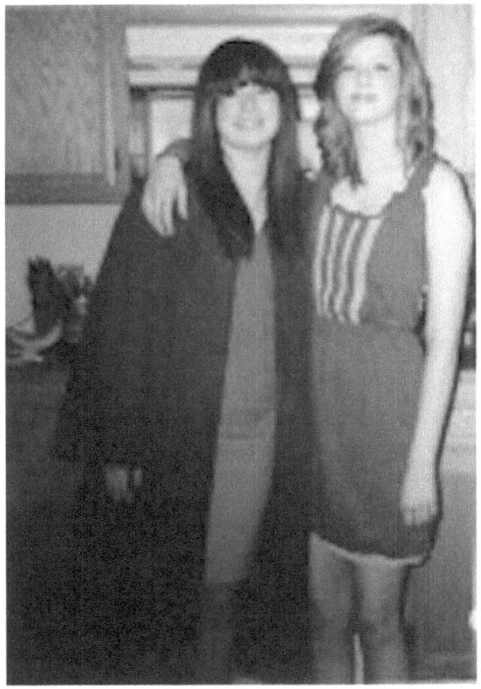

Granddaughters Tristian and Chelsea.

Left to right: (Son) Michael, Dianne (Mom), (Daughter) Rhonda, Bob (Husband), (Daughter) Candee.

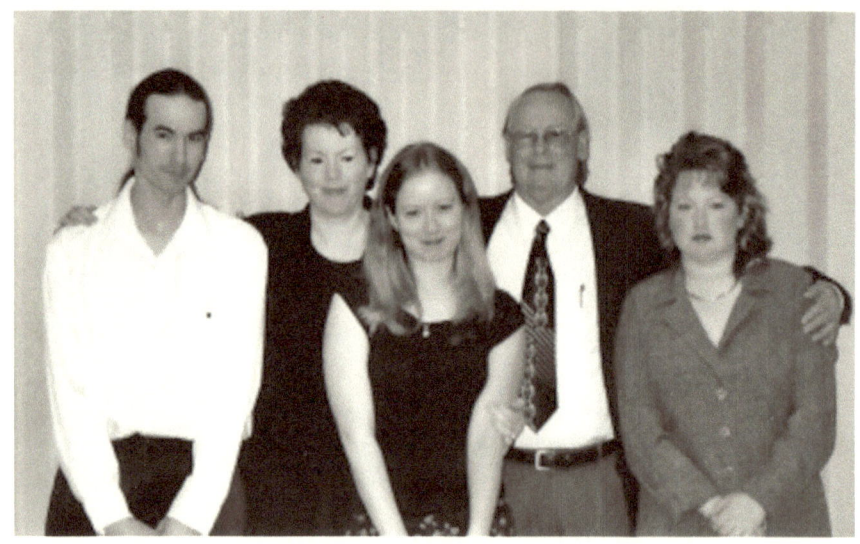

Our Family

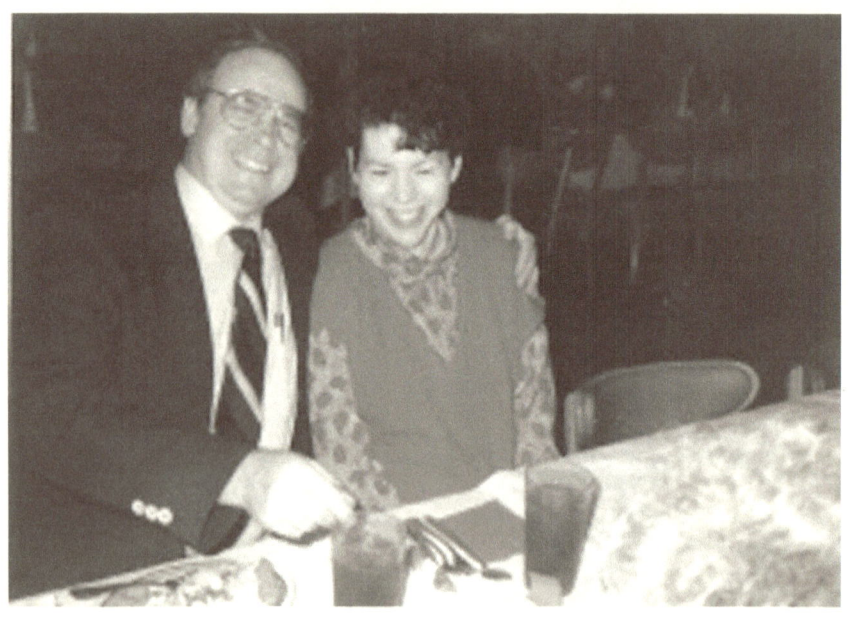

Bob and Dianne

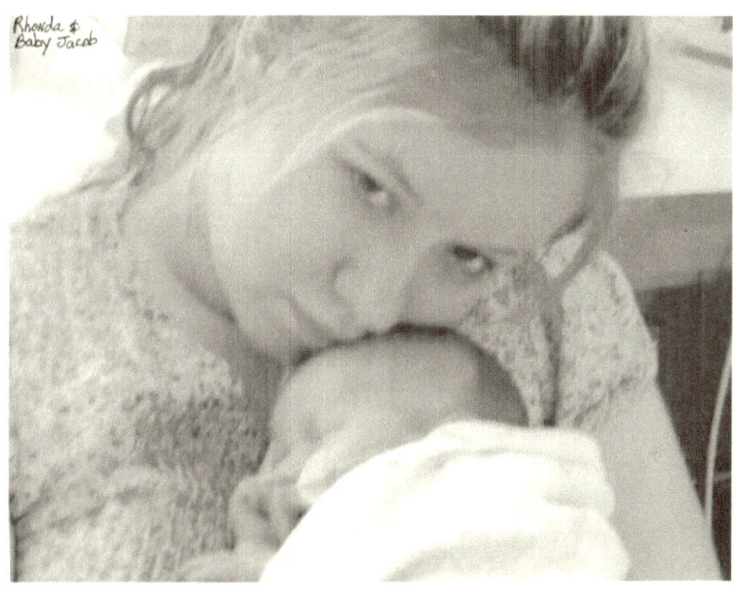
Rhonda &
Baby Jacob

www.ingramcontent.com/pod-product-compliance
Lightning Source LLC
Chambersburg PA
CBHW050336290526
45785CB00006B/2511